THE BEGINNINGS AND BENEFITS OF
ACUPUNCTURE

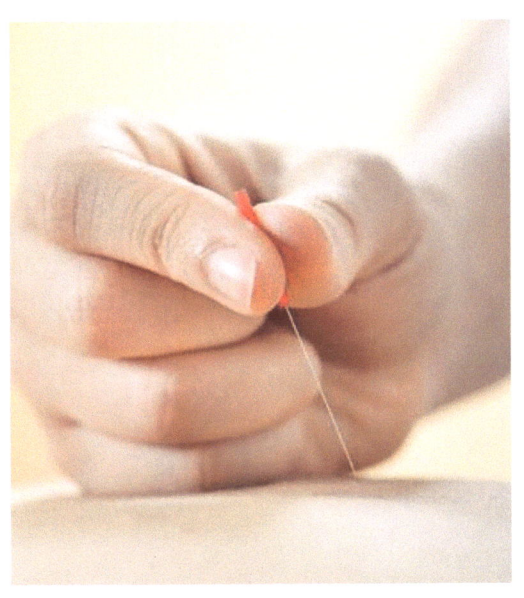

Paolo Jose de Luna

Table of Contents

Introduction

Pains and aches can have devastating effects on the quality of life, especially if they occur in various parts of the human body. If you have been struggling with them for a long time and you have no idea what to do, then this book is meant for someone like you.

In an ideal world, the human body needs to stay healthy all the time and that is why everyone is trying to stay healthy by taking the necessary steps. However, various types of pain occur frequently despite eating the right foods, exercising properly, and taking pain medication. It could just be a simple pain in the stomach, a sore on your foot, or a backache. Several factors may lead to these simple pains, but the most common cause is the pressure the body is exposed to when carrying out everyday tasks. This often happens without your knowledge, so you only realize there is a problem when you start to experience the pain.

The pressure may result from the things you do daily including the simplest ones. Depending on what you do or where you work, chances are you are likely to experience some sort of pain. If you work in an office or freelance at home, you probably sit down most of the time and this could cause back pain. You may also experience a lot of pain if your everyday work involves standing for a long time without taking a break. People who are at a higher risk of experiencing pain are those who engage in strenuous activities such as lifting or carrying heavy objects every day.

As you can see, everyone is at risk when it comes to pains and aches because of the things we do daily. These include even the simplest home and office chores. You cannot tell when the pain will occur because it can strike without a warning. Although everyone can experience some form of pain at any given moment, joint pains and backaches are more likely to occur in adults in their mid-twenties and thirties. Elderly people who are at least 70 years old are also prone to these pains.

If you realize you can no longer perform your daily duties because of pains, you should look for the appropriate solutions. Sudden muscle pains, backaches, and joint paints may have serious effects or signify an underlying health problem, so it is advisable to have them checked. The pain may result from a severe health problem that needs further advice from a professional healthcare practitioner and immediate treatment. Your doctor will carry out the necessary clinical examinations and recommend the appropriate treatment for the problem.

Of course, it is important to visit a doctor for recommendations if you are experiencing severe pain, but there are other options. Various factors may make want to use alternative treatment options that have proven to be effective over the years. The truth is that some people may not have enough money to pay for treatment in a healthcare facility. They might even lack the money needed to pay consultation fees. For these and other reasons, many people look for alternative treatment options. Luckily, there are several alternatives to choose from if you often suffer from pains and aches.

Acupuncture is one of the best treatment options for those suffering from different types of pains and aches. This treatment method has been around for many years and has proven to be an effective treatment for joint pains, back pains, and other pains. In this book, you will learn everything you need to know about acupuncture. The key areas of focus include the history of acupuncture, health benefits, application in different areas, and safety issues. As you read the book, you will learn how acupuncture works and know the right time to use this method of treatment. You will also learn about the specific steps taken by an acupuncturist and the possible side effects.

Paolo Jose de Luna

CHAPTER 1:

The History of Acupuncture

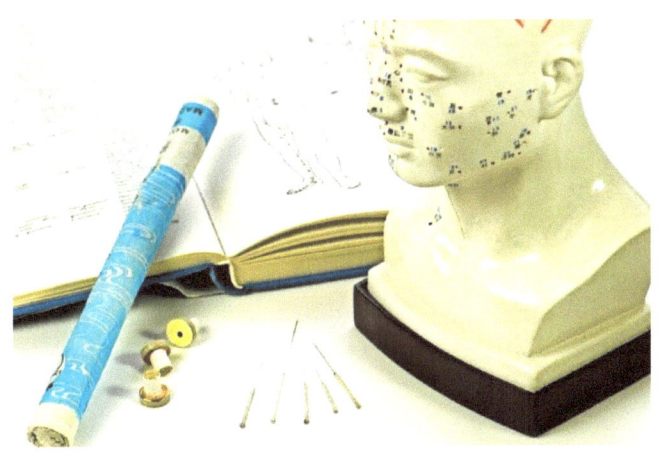

Understanding Acupuncture

Acupuncture is one of the most popular forms of alternative medicine. The Chinese were the first people to use this traditional method of treatment. Even today, acupuncture is still a major component of Chinese medicine. The practice has gained popularity over the years and spread to other parts of the world. During an acupuncture session, the practitioner or acupuncturist inserts thin needles into specific parts of the patient's body. These points are commonly known as acupuncture points or pressure points.

In some cases, an acupuncture session many involve other practices besides inserting the needles. For example, the acupuncturist may apply laser light, heat or pressure to the pressure points. Over the years, acupuncturists have used the practice to help patients with all types of health conditions. However, most of the people who benefit from the services of an acupuncturist are those experiencing pains and aches in different parts of the body.

Today, acupuncture is a common practice in clinical settings and the steps taken to treat a patient vary from one country to another. Since the traditional Chinese practice of acupuncture has no scientific basis, acupuncture is termed as a pseudoscience. In other words, this form of traditional Chinese medicine is based on practices and beliefs that are claimed to be factual and scientific but are not compatible with scientific methods.

Acupuncture History

The Chinese are famous for a wide range of health practices that have proven to be effective in treating various health problems. Therefore, it is no surprise that they were the first people to practice acupuncture. Most accounts of the practice point towards the Chinese. Just like moxibustion (the practice of burning dried mugwort on certain parts of the body), acupuncture is an ancient practice in traditional Chinese medicine.

Many theories have emerged in an attempt to explain how the Chinese discovered and began to use acupuncture to treat people. According to some historians, the *Huangdi Neijing,* which was later given the title *"The Yellow Emperor's Classic of Internal Medicine"*, was the first to document acupuncture as an organized method of diagnosing and treating certain health conditions. According to one Rheumatology article, the initial documentation of the practice dates back to 100 BC. Of course, evidence is a key factor when it comes to proving that acupuncture existed at that time.

If you are still skeptical about the origins of acupuncture and its practice, there is evidence to support the claim that the practice existed as early as 100 BC. The first significant evidence was in the form of needles, which are an important component of any acupuncture treatment session. This evidence was in the form of silver and gold needles which were found in Liu Sheng's tomb. Based on this evidence, the needles were from around 100 BC. Although the main purpose of the needles was not clear, there is a chance that they were used during acupuncture sessions.

According to another account of the history of acupuncture, it is believed that the first practice of acupuncture was recorded in the Historical Records or *Shih-Chi* in Chinese. Historians claim that these records date back to 100 BC. Also, historians claim that these historical records of the practice provided information about a practice that had already gained popularity in many areas. Based on this claim, it is possible that the Chinese were practicing acupuncture even before the 100 BCs.

As you can see, the historical account of the origins of acupuncture is based on ancient texts and that is why it is not easy to establish the exact year or date when people started to practice acupuncture. According to two academics named Buell and Ramey, the exact year the practice of acupuncture started depends on how much we can trust ancient records. Another important factor to consider when examining the origin of acupuncture is our interpretation of the practice based on the available evidence. We already know that acupuncture probably began before 100 BC. However, most of the ancient texts suggest that the practice started after 2000 BC. This makes acupuncture one of the oldest forms of traditional Chinese medicine.

Other Theories

Other theories have also tried to explain the origins and the earliest practice of acupuncture. One of the popular theories is based on the story of the iceman mummy nicknamed Ötzi. According to archeologists, the mummified corpse was at least 5,000 years old. One of the things that captured the attention of the archeologists was the various groups of tattoos (at least fifteen) on the mummified corpse. The most interesting thing about the tattoos is that they were located at pressure points where acupuncture practitioners would have placed the needles to treat a patient suffering from lower back and abdominal pain.

Based on evidence from the body, the researchers had a good reason to believe that Ötzi had experienced lower back and abdominal pains. Also, the location of the tattoos on several acupuncture points indicated that Ötzi probably used some form of acupuncture. This evidence also suggests that the practice of acupuncture may have been used in Europe and Asia in the early years of the Bronze Age.

The story of Ötzi faced criticism in *The Oxford Handbook of the History of Medicine* the major one being that it was completely based on speculation. The researchers assumed that the presence of tattoos in various pressure points meant that Ötzi had used acupuncture at some point. According to the handbook, there are low chances that acupuncture started before 2000 BC. The key argument in the book is that the practice of acupuncture is most likely to have started in the Neolithic period when the Stone Age was about to end.

At that time, it is believed that humans practiced acupuncture using sharpened stones known as *Bian shi*. The Chinese mentioned these stones in texts written during the later period. The texts talked about sharp stones known as "plen". The literal meaning of "plen" is "stone probe". Based on this meaning, it is possible that people who lived in that era used the stones to perform acupuncture. There is significant evidence from ancient Chinese texts to support this claim. A good example is the traditional Chinese text, *Huangdi Neijing*. According to the text, it is believed that people in ancient China used sharp stones to treat health problems. People would also place the stones near or on the patient's body for healing purposes. This is probably because the stones were short and not sharp enough to penetrate the body.

Acupuncture may not be the only reason why people used stones. It is believed that people used sharp stones to perform various medical procedures such as draining pus from a growth. The user would puncture the growth with the sharp end of the stone. The Mawangdui texts also played an important role in explaining the other uses of sharp stones in addition to their possible use in acupuncture sessions. According to the texts, the pointed stones were probably used in the second century BC to open abscesses. At that time, the stones were mainly used for moxibustion rather than acupuncture.

According to *The Oxford Handbook of the History of Medicine*, people who existed at that time used the stones for bloodletting. The practice of bloodletting involves withdrawing blood from the patient's body to prevent or treat health conditions. People who practiced bloodletting held that cutting the patient's skin would promote life energy flow by clearing blockages. Life energy is known as "chi" or "qi", which is pronounced as "chee". The available evidence shows that bloodletting probably existed before acupuncture and contributed to the practice of acupuncture. The Chinese also believed in spiritual methods of healing, Yin Yang, and other early beliefs that played an important role in the inception of acupuncture.

In another theory, the historians Joseph Needham and Lu Gwei-djen differed with the aforementioned historians about the exact date when the practice of acupuncture started. According to the two historians, a large percentage of the available evidence showed that the practice started around 600 BC. At the time, those who practiced acupuncture were probably using other locally available materials. For example, if the Chinese practiced acupuncture during the era of the Shang Dynasty (1766 – 1122 BC), chances are they were using organic materials like bamboo, sharpened stones, and thorns.

Needham and Gwe-djen based their theory on some pictograms and hieroglyphs dating back to that era. According to the evidence gathered by the historians, the people of that era were using moxibustion and acupuncture to help those suffering from health problems. The reason why the historians claim that acupuncture involved the use of organic materials is that the Chinese were unlikely to make needles from the materials that were available at that time. However, their argument was based on speculation and it is not clear whether they were right or wrong.

Apart from bamboo, stones, and thorns, it is also said that those who practiced acupuncture during the early days probably used other materials. For instance, if acupuncture started in 600 BC, it is possible that the early practitioners used bronze to make needles for the practice. Other materials that would be perfect for making needles at that time include gold, silver, copper, and tin. However, the latter materials were unlikely to be common at that time. Perhaps they were only used occasionally and in rare situations.

As the years went by, the ancient Chinese learned to make needles using other materials. For example, Needham and Gwe-djen believed that steel replaced the other materials when humans discovered effective steel production methods. People discovered that steel was better than other material because it was durable and they could use to make fine needles. While Needham and Gwe-djen noted that the ancient humans were using ancient materials like bamboo, sharpened stones, and thorns to make needles for acupuncture, they also claimed that people used these tools to perform other tasks.

Documents believed to be from 198 BC were discovered in the tomb of Ma-Wang-Diu did not mention the practice of acupuncture. If we base our argument on the text, then it is unlikely that the ancient Chinese who lived at that time were practicing acupuncture.

Other Beliefs

Based on what we have learned so far, it is evident that different historians had different beliefs regarding when the practice of acupuncture started. There are many conflicting beliefs probably because the different schools of thought were competing to provide the best explanation of when people started to use acupuncture as a disease prevention and treatment method. According to evidence found in some early texts, the early humans used acupuncture for bloodletting purposes.

Other ancient texts combined the idea of spiritual energy or chi with the practice of bloodletting. However, these ideas changed over the years and humans shifted from the idea of bloodletting to the idea of puncturing certain parts of the human body. They also shifted to the idea of balancing the body's positive (Yin) and negative (Yang) energies. Yin and Yang is a concept of dualism in traditional Chinese philosophy. It describes how seemingly opposite forces or aspects of the human body may be interdependent, complementary or interconnected.

Dr. David Ramey asserts that no single theory was predominantly used as a standard because of the lack of scientific knowledge in the field of medicine at that time. One good reason is that dissecting a dead body was not allowed in China. This and other factors made it difficult to develop the basic knowledge of anatomy.

It is widely believed that the ancient Chinese discovered the practice of puncturing specific parts of the body to prevent and cure certain health problems. However, there is insufficient information about when humans discovered the specific pressure or acupuncture points on the human body. Based on information from Pien Chhio's autobiography, which was written somewhere between 400 and 500 BC, humans would insert needles into specific parts of the body. According to Bian Que, the top part of the skull was a single pressure point known as the point of hundred meetings.

Other texts that were written around 156 BC – 186 BC documented beliefs in life energy channels. These channels are commonly known as meridians. Beliefs in the flow of energy through these passageways later became an important part of acupuncture beliefs. In acupuncture, meridians are simply the pathways through which energy flows throughout the human body.

According to Buell and Ramey, the modern-day practice of acupuncture is based on the theories and practices introduced at around 100 BC in the *Huangdi Neijing*. This includes the idea of manipulating energy flow (chi) in the body. The process involves manipulating a large network within the patient's body. The network consists of acu-tracts where the acupoints are located. Most of the people who practice acupuncture today use the same acupoint names as described in the *Huangdi Neijing*.

Over the years, more documents detailing new acupoints were published. Most of the acupoints targeted during acupuncture sessions today had already been identified and named by 300 AD.

CHAPTER 2:

The Use of Acupuncture in Ancient China

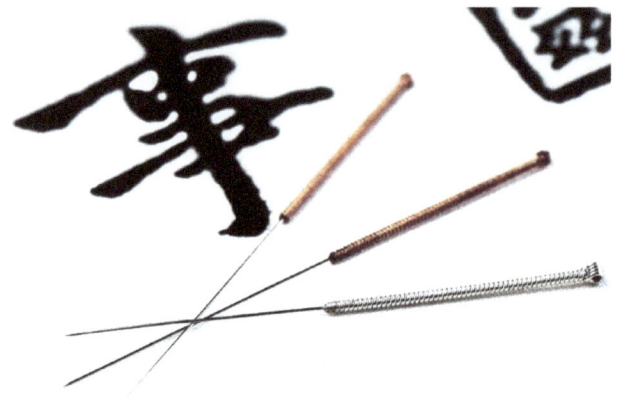

One of the best ways to understand the history and practice of acupuncture in China is to look at evidence from ancient books. Books with information about acupuncture practices were written and published as early as the 1st century AD. Recognized acupuncture practitioners and experts also started to emerge at that time. The *Zhen Jiu Jia Yi Jing* is considered to be the earliest book that recorded the practice of acupuncture. Based on the available evidence, the book was probably published around the 200s. The Director of Medical Services for China also wrote another influential book titled *Yu Kuei Chen Ching*. However, the book has not been preserved.

The practice of acupuncture in ancient China has also been explained using charts and diagrams. Sun Simiao is one of the writers who created acupuncture related charts and diagrams in the 600s. The charts and diagrams played an important role in creating a standardized system for grouping the various acupuncture points on the human body. The standardized system was known as the *thung shen tshun fa*. Sun Simiao realized that the diagrams had some discrepancies, so he decided to create the "relative inches" system that uses a person's size to find acupuncture points using a standardized procedure. One way to find an individual's "inch" for acupuncture purposes was to use their middle finger length.

As time went by, the practice of acupuncture gained popularity in China spreading to different parts of the country. The paper production industry was also growing at an incredible rate due to technological improvements. As a result, the ancient Chinese were able to write and publish more books about acupuncture treatment. The Imperial Medical College and the Imperial Medical Service began to support acupuncture, so the practice became more popular than before. Another significant development in China was the establishment of colleges for medical students in all provinces. Members of the public were also exposed to the practice through stories of noble people who had benefited from the services of prominent acupuncturists.

Today, most of the practices used by acupuncture practitioners had already gained popularity during the era of the Ming Dynasty (1368-1644 AD) when *The Great Compendium of Acupuncture and Moxibustion* was printed. However, there were significant differences in terms of the tools used to perform acupuncture. For example, the needles used at that time were thicker than the ones used today. The earliest needles also caused more infections than the modern-day needles.

People had interesting explanations of the possible causes of infections during acupuncture sessions. Some people believed that infections occurred because acupuncture practitioners used the wrong needles and followed the wrong procedures. They did not know that the infections occurred because acupuncture providers failed to sterilize the needles.

After realizing what was happening, people decided to find a way to prevent infections during acupuncture sessions. Later, acupuncture practitioners realized that they could sterilize needles by heating them in flames or boiling water. In some cases, acupuncturists would perform the procedure using hot needles to create a cauterizing sensation. The *Chen Chiu Ta Chheng* (1601) recommended more than 9 needles because 9 was believed to be a magical number in traditional Chinese beliefs.

Acupuncturists also began to promote a wide range of beliefs regarding the effectiveness of acupuncture. For example, some claimed that the effectiveness of the practice depended on time (day/night), seasons, and the lunar phase in the early years of the 1st century AD. Others based their arguments on *Yün Chhi Hsüeh* or Yin-Yang science claiming that curing illnesses depended on the proper alignment of earthly (ti) and heavenly (thien) forces. These forces were related to the sun and moon cycles. At that time, there were many belief systems based on rotating earthly and celestial bodies that aligned at specific times. People also started to believe that some health problems were caused by a Yin-Yang imbalance.

People noticed that some health problems were corresponding to certain weather and spiritual conditions. Such health problems were mainly considered to be heart problems or fever. There was also the belief that the body functioned on a specific rhythm. For this reason, the practice of acupuncture was used to correct the rhythm and make it more effective by placing acupuncture needles at specific parts of the body. According to Gwei-djen and Needham, acupuncture practitioners depicted these random predictions in sophisticated charts. Several terminologies were created based on predictions of the time when certain events occurred.

In the final years of the Song Dynasty (1279 AD), acupuncture was almost losing its status in China. Since then, the practice lost its popularity for hundreds of years and was considered to be a less prestigious practice like moxibustion, midwifery, alchemy, and shamanism. The practice of acupuncture in China faced more challenges in the 1700s because many people had started to believe in scientific research more than superstitious beliefs.

A history of medicine in China was published by 1757 describing acupuncture as one of the lost arts. In 1822, a decree was signed by the emperor to exclude acupuncture practices from the Imperial Medical Institute. According to the Chinese Emperor, gentlemen-scholars could not practice acupuncture because it was unfit for them.

The practice of acupuncture continued to lose its popularity in China and many people started to associate it with illiterate practitioners who were considered to be lower-class citizens. After some time, the practice was reinstated but was later prohibited in 1929. By that time, Western medical practices that were based on scientific research had already started to gain popularity in many countries including China.

While the practice of acupuncture was declining in China, it was gaining popularity in various countries at the same time. By 1949, acupuncture had started to gain popularity in China during the era of Mao Tse-Tung and the communist revolution. During the same period, many Eastern health practices were acknowledged as what is now known as traditional Chinese medicine.

How Acuncture Was Received by the International Community

According to information from various sources, it is believed that Korea was the first Asian country to practice acupuncture. One Korean legend tells the story of Emperor Dangun who played an important role in developing the practice of acupuncture. However, chances are that the people of Korea learned about acupuncture from a colonial territory in 514 AD. By the sixth century, acupuncture was already a popular practice in Korea. After reaching Korea, it was brought into Vietnam between the eight and the ninth century.

By the 9th century AD, Vietnam had started to trade with other countries including China and Japan. As a result, the people of Vietnam learned how to practice acupuncture. By 219 BC, medical missionaries from Korea and China were sent to promote traditional medical practices in Japan. At around 553, many people from Korea and China were selected to restructure medical training in Japan and that is when acupuncture was included in Japan's medical education. The students then traveled from Japan to China to establish acupuncture as a division of the medical system in China. Acupuncture became one of the 5 divisions of China's medical system.

Acupuncture later became popular in European countries during the 2nd half of the seventieth century. At that time, Dutch East Indie Company's surgeon-general met acupuncture practitioners from Japan and China. He later encouraged European countries to carry out more research on the practice of acupuncture. France was one of the first countries to accept acupuncture due to the efforts of Jesuit missionaries. In the 16th century, the missionaries played an important role in bringing acupuncture to clinics in France. Although some details are still debatable, Louis Berlioz is widely recognized as the first French doctor to experiment with the procedure. Sources claim that he first experimented with acupuncture in 1810 and published the results in 1816.

The practice of acupuncture started to capture the attention of Britons and Americans at the beginning of the 20th century. However, those who practiced acupuncture in the west abandoned the traditional beliefs associated with the practice. Some of the things they abandoned included the idea of spiritual energy, moon cycles, sun cycles, and the rhythm of the body. There were also significant differences between anatomical designs from the west and anatomical designs from the east. For example, spiritual energy diagrams from both regions had notable differences with regard to energy flow. Acupuncture practitioners based their practice on the notion of inserting needles into the human body to stimulate the nerves.

The media also played a crucial role in popularizing the practice of acupuncture in America. In 1971, one reporter wrote an article for NY Times to let Americans and the world at large learn about his experiences after receiving acupuncture in China. The article prompted more investigations leading to more acupuncture activities in the US. Later on, more people and organizations began to support the use of acupuncture in America. For example, the National Institute of Health (NIH) started to support the practice for certain types of health conditions. This was an important step even though the NIH only supported acupuncture for a few health conditions.

People in Western countries interpreted acupuncture based on beliefs in various trigger points. They believed that these trigger points could trigger pain. The trigger points were the same acupuncture points identified by the Chinese, but people from the west were using a different system of beliefs. The Dutch physician William ten Rhiine published the first detailed Western treatise in 1683. The physician had been working at Dejima (Dutch trading post) in Nagasaki for 2 years.

Many countries had already accepted the practice of acupuncture by the 19th century. At that time, some ancient beliefs of the practice were abandoned and people interpreted drawings of acu-tracts as drawings of blood veins in the human body. Many acupuncturists started to use needle clusters in the early years of the 20th century. The needle clusters were simultaneously hammered into the patient's body using slight taps. Acupuncture practitioners also started using other techniques such as passing electric currents through the needles after insertion. Some acupuncturists would also leave the needles in for several days. Those who practiced acupuncture believed that it worked by stimulating the nerves. Later on, acupuncturists started to pay attention to the ear.

CHAPTER 3:

Acupuncture in Different Parts of the World Today

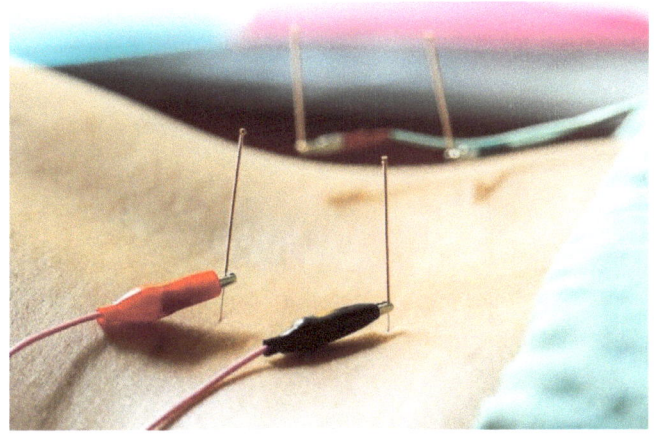

China

The field of healthcare experienced significant growth in the twentieth century because of technological changes that led to the development of new types of medicines. Western culture spread rapidly to other parts of the world and China was one of the first countries to use Western medicine. By 1929, the people of China were prohibited from using acupuncture and other traditional medical practices that were practiced in the country at that time. However, these practices were later allowed in 1949 because of the efforts of the Communist Party. After the reinstallation of traditional medicine practices in China, many conflicting theories and beliefs about traditional medicine turned into what is now known as traditional Chinese medicine or TCM.

When the people of China were allowed to continue using traditional Chinese medicine, acupuncture gained popularity and became a part of the healthcare system. Modern hospitals started to offer acupuncture services and research organizations that focused on the practice of acupuncture emerged in the 1950s.

Acupuncture and other forms of traditional Chinese medicine faced a lot of resistance before they became popular in China. A good example is what happened when the Civil War was just starting in China. At that time, leaders of the famous Communist Party ridiculed and were not willing to accept traditional Chinese medicine. According to the leaders, practices like acupuncture were irrational, backward, and based on superstitions. The leaders and members of the party claimed that they had embraced science, so the practice of acupuncture and other forms of TCM did not align with the party's scientific view of medical practices. They believed science was the future.

Mao Zedong was the Communist Party's leader at that time. The decision to use medicine that was only based on science was reversed during his tenure. Members of the party were encouraged to support pharmacology as well as traditional Chinese medicine because both options were useful and could be explored to a greater level for the benefit of the people of China.

One of the problems experienced by the Chinese when Mao Zedong was in power was the lack of medical practitioners with experience in modern healthcare practices. Under the leadership of Mao Zedong, the Communist Party responded to this problem by accepting and reviving acupuncture as a treatment method. However, the theory of acupuncture had to be rewritten for economic, political, and logistical reasons. The main goal of rewriting the theory was to make it easy for the people of China to receive the healthcare services they needed at that time.

Mao Zedong went to the extent of proclaiming that Chinese medicine was scientific. However, the truth is that Chinese medicine was based on Marxism or historical materialism. Marxists tried to oppose superstitious practices rather than Western practices based on empirical investigations of nature. There was conflict even after rewriting the theory of traditional Chinese medicine, so Mao tried to solve the problem using a different approach. He insisted that the theory needed to be rewritten, which happened in the 1950s. His political response to the problem aimed to address the existing discord between traditional Chinese medicine and scientific medicine.

Mao also wanted to rectify conventional and materialistic thoughts of the type of medicine used by Western doctors. Despite doing all these things, Mao Zedong did not use TCM because he did not believe in it. He only proclaimed it to the members of the public.

United States

The practice of acupuncture was not recognized in the United States of America until 1972. This was a special year because Richard Nixon, the US president at that time, had traveled to China where he learned about acupuncture. During his visit, the president had an incredible experience during a surgical procedure. He had the privilege of watching doctors perform a major surgical procedure while the patient was awake during the entire process. According to reports, the doctors allegedly used acupuncture instead of anesthesia after undergoing the procedure.

After the procedure, reports indicated that something was not right about the entire procedure. For example, it was discovered that the procedure was performed on patients who were extremely intolerant to pain. Additionally, reports showed that the patients received indoctrination before undergoing the procedure. This means they were instructed to accept certain beliefs.

Another problem with these demonstration medical procedures was that the patients received morphine regularly. Morphine is a type of pain medication that acts on the central nervous system to decrease the feeling of pain. It can be used to reduce chronic or acute pain. The drug was administered using an intravenous drip. People who were watching the procedure were told that the drip contained only nutrients and fluids. There was also another case of a patient who was undergoing open-heart surgery. According to sources, the patient had received three different types of powerful sedatives and heavy injections of anesthetics. This explains why the patient managed to stay awake during the procedure without showing any signs of pain.

Although acupuncture had already gained popularity in China when these events were unfolding, it took some time before it was officially recognized in Western countries. The first significant event which helped popularize the practice was when a NY Times reporter named James Reston went to Beijing in 1971. The reporter received acupuncture to treat pain after an operation and decided to write about his experience in the newspaper. His report played an important role in exposing the practice of acupuncture and the US started to recognize it as an alternative method of treatment.

In 1972, the US established the first, legally-recognized acupuncture center in Washington DC. This marked the beginning of acupuncture treatment in the United States and many people started to look for the services of acupuncturists. Up to 1,000 patients visited the newly established acupuncture center between 1973 and 1974. At the same time, the Internal Revenue Service (IRS) acknowledged acupuncture as an expense that could be deducted. This was a major step in the history of acupuncture in the US and one of the reasons why the practice has gained popularity in America and other parts of the world.

Studies on the number of acupuncture users in the US have revealed a significant increase over the years. According to studies conducted in the 1990s, the number of people who were using acupuncture treatment was less than 1%. However, studies conducted in the 2010s have shown that there are over 14 million acupuncture users in America. This is enough evidence to prove that Americans have fully embraced the practice of acupuncture.

CHAPTER 4:

Acupuncture in Other Parts of the World

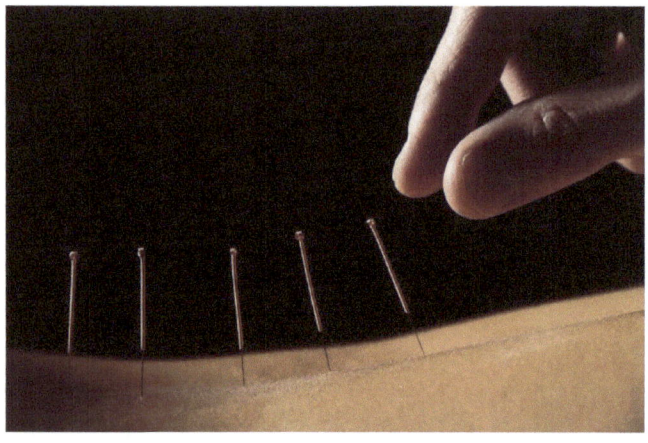

Based on what we know so far, acupuncture is a popular practice in China and has gained popularity in the United States. Other countries have also followed the footsteps of China and the US. Some of the places where acupuncture is popular nowadays include Europe, Australia, and all Nordic countries (Denmark, Iceland, Sweden, Finland, and Norway). However, the practice is less popular in Finland. Today, acupuncture has gained popularity in many European countries as a form of alternative medicine. Here are some of the countries where acupuncture is a common practice.

United Kingdom

The United Kingdom is one of the most popular places where acupuncture is widely used as an alternative treatment method. According to data collected in 2009, about four million people received acupuncture treatment in the UK that year. Those living in the UK can find and receive acupuncture services in various places including hospitals and pain clinics. Today, the National Institute for Health and Care Excellence (NICE) recommends acupuncture for treating tension-type headaches and migraines. Some GP practices also offer integrated healthcare that includes acupuncture although this is not a popular service.

Australia

The people of Australia started to fully recognize acupuncture in the 1880s as a form of alternative and complementary medicine. However, the practice was introduced to Australians by the first Chinese immigrant workers in the 1850s. The number of registered acupuncture practitioners in Australia has increased since the 1990s reaching nearly 4,000 practitioners in the year 2014. According to data collected in 2004, about one in ten adult Australians used acupuncture treatment that year. Nowadays, Australians can receive acupuncture from acupuncturists or general practitioners with solid training in acupuncture.

Germany

Germany is another country that has adopted acupuncture as an alternative treatment method. According to a study conducted in 2007, the number of acupuncture users in Germany increased by 20% that year. This happened after some trials revealed that acupuncture was effective for certain applications. The trials made it possible for Germans who wanted to use acupuncture to make insurance claims. Public health insurers included acupuncture service in health insurance, but they only agreed to cover knee osteoarthritis and chronic back pain. They refused to offer coverage for migraines and tension headache for reasons that were considered to be socio-political. Other health insurers stopped offering coverage for acupuncture.

It was difficult to convince public health insurers that acupuncture could treat other health conditions better than the usual treatment methods used in the country. Based on results from the placebo subjects, researchers were not convinced that placebo therapy was effective. In the year 2011, more than 1 million Germans used acupuncture treatment. When it comes to gender differences in the use of acupuncture in Germany, a study conducted by some health insurers shows that more than 60% of Germans who use acupuncture treatment are women.

Japan

According to some experts, about 25% of people in Japan will use acupuncture treatment at some point. Despite the relatively large number of acupuncture users and practitioners in the country, public health insurers are reluctant to cover acupuncture treatment. However, there are a few exceptions including low back pain, neuralgia, neck sprain, rheumatoid arthritis, frozen shoulder, and cervico-branchial syndrome, only when the patient gets the appropriate document from a physician. Overall, only a few healthcare providers are willing to recommend acupuncture to their patients in Japan.

The truth is that it is hard for acupuncture users to get help from Japanese public health insurers. Nevertheless, those with the appropriate skills in acupuncture can obtain a license and practice in their own clinics. License for acupuncture is a national qualification and those looking for one are required to complete a three-year program in an accredited vocational school or a four-year program in an accredited university.

Research findings have shown that most Japanese users of acupuncture are elderly people with limited education. According to one study, about 50% of acupuncture users in Japan were likely to use this form of treatment in the future. However, 37% of the users said they would not use this type of treatment again.

Switzerland

Switzerland is one of the places where acupuncture is a popular form of alternative medicine. according to research, there has been a significant increase in the number of users since 2004. Since healthcare professionals in Switzerland are regulated by individual cantons or regions, licenses for acupuncture practitioners are issued by the cantons, and very different conditions apply. Medical doctors can offer acupuncture services and use Chinese herbs in all cantons. If doctors want to be reimbursed by the country's compulsory health insurance, they need to have a certificate that requires a minimum training time of 360 hours in Chinese herbal medicine and acupuncture.

Scientific Research

Over the years, the practice of acupuncture has attracted the attention of scientists and researchers in the field of medicine. Active research on the practice started towards the end of the 20th century. By the year 2006, many researchers had already carried out various scientific studies. The key areas of research included the basis of acupuncture and its effectiveness in preventing or treating certain health problems. Although acupuncture is a popular treatment method in today's field of medicine, it is still a controversial practice.

The practice of acupuncture has also attracted the attention of people in the TV industry and has featured in documentaries. A good example is the "Alternative Medicine" documentary produced by BBC. The documentary is about a patient who allegedly underwent open-heart surgery using acupuncture as a form of anesthesia. However, it was later discovered that the doctors had combined a variety of weak anesthetics. It turned out that the mixture was more powerful than the individual drugs used to create the mixture. The program faced a lot of criticism for its fanciful explanation of the findings.

Overall, the people of China are famous for using acupuncture as a disease prevention and treatment method. Regardless of where they live on the planet, the Chinese still believe in the benefits of acupuncture and consider the practice to be an important aspect of their culture.

CHAPTER 5:

Health Benefits and Side Effects of Acupuncture

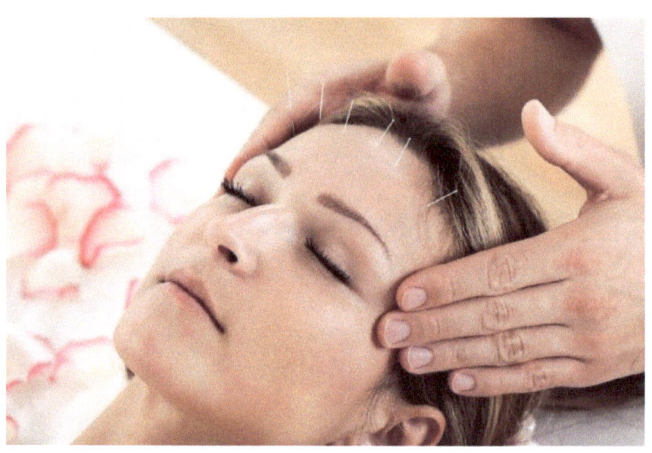

Now that we have learned a lot about the history and application of acupuncture in healthcare practices, it is time to find out the different types of patients who can benefit from the services of an acupuncturist. According to the NIH (National Institute of Health), the Consensus Development Program developed in 1977 aims at assessing health technology. One of the program's key goals is to organize major conferences to produce technology assessment and consensus statements on debatable healthcare issues. This includes controversial issues that are important to patients, healthcare providers, and members of the public.

According to a statement issued by the NIH on 3-5 November 1997, acupuncture is a recognized and widely used therapeutic intervention in the US. Although many researchers have tried to find out whether acupuncture is an effective treatment method, the results have been equivocal due to various factors. These factors include the size of the sample, study design and many more.

Researchers have also faced other challenges that have made it more difficult to assess the potential usefulness of acupuncture. One of the reasons why the practice of acupuncture is a complex issue is that there have been significant problems with controls. For instance, researchers have faced problems when using sham and placebo acupuncture groups.

Health Problems That Can Be Treated Using Acupuncture

Despite the aforementioned challenges, some studies have produced promising results. For example, some studies have revealed that acupuncture is an efficient method when used by adult patients after undergoing surgery. Research findings have also shown that adults who vomit and experience pain or nausea after dental surgical procedures can benefit from acupuncture.

According to research, those suffering from drug addiction, headache, stroke rehabilitation, tennis elbow, carpal tunnel syndrome, lower back pain, myofascial pain, fibromyalgia, menstrual cramps, and osteoarthritis may benefit from acupuncture. Other people who might benefit from the procedure are those suffering from chest pain, arthritis, asthma, labor pain, depression, and other psychological problems. Those suffering from these problems may benefit if acupuncture is combined with other treatments or used as an alternative treatment option. Acupuncture can also be used if the patient is using a comprehensive program to manage a health problem.

Although researchers have experienced several challenges trying to find out the efficiency of acupuncture, basic research has started to clarify the treatment method's mechanisms when used by patients with different health problems. Some of the mechanisms highlighted in basic research include the production of opioids as well as peptides in the patient's nervous system. Research has also focused on the effects of acupuncture on the functions of neuroendocrine systems. Overall, research has supported plausible mechanisms and more research is needed to support the effects of acupuncture when used to help patients with different types of health problems. The available evidence is still encouraging and that is why many people are using acupuncture treatment today.

When it comes to the adoption of acupuncture in today's treatment modalities, the practice is still in the early stages of adoption due to various reasons. The first reason is the issue of training. In most countries, people who want to practice acupuncture are required to undergo training to avoid legal issues. Similarly, those with intentions of practicing acupuncture need to obtain the appropriate license from the relevant organizations. The other reason why the practice of acupuncture is still in the initial stages is the issue of reimbursement. These factors need proper clarification for acupuncture treatment to move to the next level. Researchers should also conduct more research to assess the value of acupuncture when combined with conventional medicine in the clinical setting. Apart from evaluating its clinical values, it is also important to assess its physiology.

CHAPTER 6:

Safety and Side Effects of Acupuncture

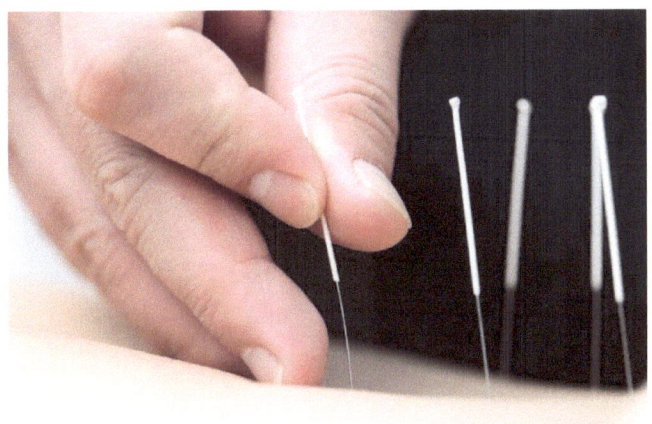

Just like any other procedure, the practice of acupuncture is associated with various safety issues as well as side effects that may have serious effects on the patient. When it comes to safety, those performing or undertaking the procedure need to keep several factors in mind. However, it is important to know that acupuncture is generally considered to be a safe procedure when performed by a certified acupuncturist or medical doctor.

One way to ensure you are safe in the hands of an acupuncture practitioner is to ensure they have obtained the necessary license. You should also make sure that your service provider has the required training. Even as you look for licensing and training information, make sure the practitioner follows the appropriate guidelines. However, keep in mind that acupuncture may be performed by unlicensed individuals in certain countries.

Other safety issues relate to what might happen after undergoing the procedure. For example, the patient may develop an infection after the procedure although such cases are rare. Since an acupuncture procedure involves inserting needles into the patient's body, an infection may occur if the needles are not sterilized. The best thing about licensed practitioners is that they know what they should do to promote hygiene and reduce the risk of infecting patients. For example, they are required to get rid of needles immediately after the procedure.

To avoid infections, acupuncture users should not share needles. Once you enter the room, confirm that your acupuncturist will use a new set of sterilized needles to avoid infections during the procedure. The same should happen when you come for another procedure to minimize the risk of infections and other transmissible health conditions.

If you are still not sure about your safety and overall wellbeing before an acupuncture session, it is advisable to consult your physician. A good doctor will let you know the risks you face if you are suffering from a certain health problem and you want to use acupuncture. Even if you are not suffering from any health problem, it is important to tell your physician. The key point is to know all the possible risks before using the services of an acupuncturist.

Patients also need to know the possible side effects of using acupuncture. Acupuncture practitioners insert needles into the patient's body. This is a dangerous procedure even when performed by an experienced acupuncturist or doctor. Accidental injury is the obvious risk when using needles to pierce the patient's body. If the needle is placed in the wrong part of the body or inserted too deep into the body, it can damage some organs. Most of the injuries reported by acupuncture users are accidental lung punctures. If the lungs are punctured during an acupuncture session, the patient may suffer from pneumothorax. This problem occurs when the punctured lung collapses and may have serious effects on the patient.

There is also a significant link between safety problems and side effects when using acupuncture. As mentioned earlier, improperly sterilized or unsterilized needles can cause infections, which can be categorized as side effects of acupuncture. Viral hepatitis is a common type of infection that can be acquired during acupuncture treatment sessions. The virus affects the patient's liver and may cause a serious infection. Other possible side effects when using acupuncture treatment include bacterial infections at the various points where the needles are inserted and injury to the nervous system.

Just like some safety issues, some of the side effects of acupuncture relate to training and poor hygiene. For this reason, it is important to make sure your service provider uses new, sterilized needles and works in a clean environment. A licensed practitioner has the appropriate license and follows the recommended procedures to reduce the risk of having side effects.

CHAPTER 7:

A Typical Acupuncture Procedure

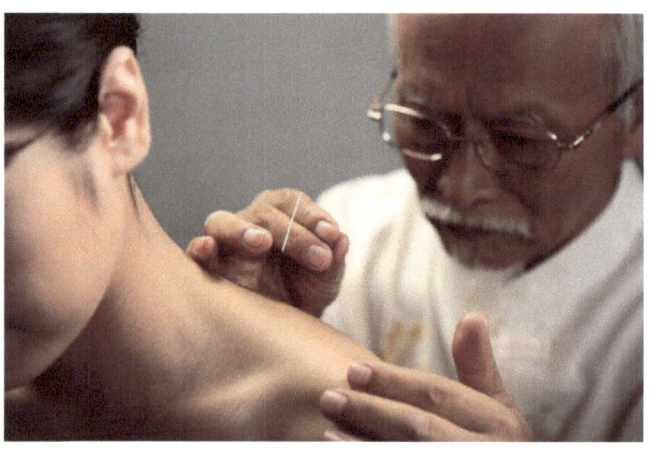

Before a typical acupuncture session, the acupuncturist will ask you to complete a health history. He or she may ask you questions about different aspects of your life including health problems, sleep, stress levels, the food you eat, and other lifestyle habits. Your acupuncturist may also want to know something about your emotions, appetite, and response to changes in the environment. Other areas which the acupuncturist might be interested in include your voice, complexion, and appearance. He or she may also take your pulse to know its strength, rhythm, and quality. If you are experiencing pain, the acupuncturist will perform a physical assessment of your body and ask questions about the pain. Overall, the acupuncturist will want to know your health status before the session begins.

After the initial assessment of your body, the next step is to look for pressure points where the flow of chi may be blocked. Each pressure point is related to specific bodily functions and health problems. The acupuncture practitioner will examine your muscles and bones to find landmarks or the right places to insert the needles. Once the practitioner finds the appropriate places to insert the needles, he or she will let you know the general site of the planned treatment. You may be required to remove some of your clothing and use a sheet, towel, or gown. Your acupuncturist will then ask you to lie down on a padded table to receive the treatment.

The provider will then start the actual procedure by inserting the needles into the identified areas. The treatment process involves the following steps:

- **Inserting the needles** – The acupuncturist will insert the needles into your body to various depths depending on what he or she thinks needs to be done to restore energy flow. Acupuncture needles are thin, so you are unlikely to experience discomfort during insertion. In most cases, acupuncturists use between 5 and 20 needles in one session.
- **Manipulating the needles** – Once the needles are in the right place, the practitioner may manipulate them. This process involves moving or twirling the needles. The practitioner may also apply mild electrical pulses or heat to the needles.
- **Removing the needles** – A typical acupuncture session lasts for about 10 to 20 minutes as you lie down on the table. However, some acupuncture treatments may take up to 60 minutes, especially the first acupuncture session. Once the session is over, the practitioner will gently remove the needles.

After the first session, the acupuncturist may ask you to come back several times to achieve the best results and complete treatment. In terms of results, every acupuncture practitioner is different, so you can expect different results from different practitioners.

Additional Techniques

Your acupuncture provider may use other techniques depending on what he or she thinks is best for you. Here are some of the common techniques that your provider might use during the session:

- **Cupping** – This procedure involves placing cups on the patient's skin to create a suction effect. In traditional Chinese medicine, cupping relieves stagnation of chi and blood.
- **Herbs** – During an acupuncture session, your provider may give you Chinese herbs in the form of tea, capsules or tablets.
- **Moxibustion** – Moxibustion involves the use of heated sticks from dried herbs. The sticks are placed near the needles to stimulate and keep the acupuncture points warm.
- **Electroacupuncture** – When using this acupuncture technique, the acupuncturist passes a small electric current between pairs of needles. Some acupuncturists claim that this practice can restore the patient's health and overall wellbeing. It is mostly used to treat pain.
- **Laser acupuncture** – As the name suggests, laser acupuncture involves the use of laser. The practitioner uses low-intensity, non-thermal laser irradiation to stimulate acupuncture points.

- **Auricular or ear acupuncture** – This acupuncture technique involves inserting needles into predetermined points on the external ear. Your acupuncturist may use it for addictions, weight loss, anxiety, and smoking cessation.

How it Feels

If you have never used acupuncture and you are ready to start your first session, you probably want to know how it feels. When the practitioner is inserting acupuncture needles into the various acupuncture points, you may experience little discomfort. However, most people do not feel any discomfort when the practitioner is inserting the needles. Overall, there is usually no discomfort when the acupuncturist is inserting the needles. Many patients say acupuncture does not hurt, but the areas where the needles are inserted may tingle, itch, feel numb, or become slightly sore. If you experience any of these feelings, it is believed that the acupuncturist has accessed the flow of energy or chi in your body.

After an acupuncture session, some people feel relaxed while others feel rejuvenated. However, some people may not respond to this form of treatment. If there are no significant changes several weeks after treatment, you may want to try a different treatment method. It is also important to conduct your doctor for advice. Hopefully, the procedure will work for you.

How it Works

Those who practice acupuncture claim that it stimulates your body's ability to overcome or resist diseases by rectifying imbalances. The needles stimulate the body to produce chemicals that are needed to eliminate or reduce painful sensations. According to acupuncturists, the human body has hundreds of acu-points or acupuncture points along 14 major meridians. As explained earlier in this book, meridians are the channels responsible for carrying energy or chi. It is believed that illnesses occur because of an imbalance of energy when the chi is disrupted. Therefore, the main purpose of acupuncture is to rectify this energy disruption to remove blockages to promote energy flow.

Various theories have emerged to explain how acupuncture works. According to one theory, the needles stimulate sensory neurons and muscles. The stimulated neurons then send a message to the CNS, which constitutes of the spinal cord and the brain. Once the CNS receives the message, endorphins and other neurotransmitters are released. Endorphins are natural pain killers and neurotransmitters are the chemicals responsible for modifying nerve impulses. The endorphins block pain messages from reaching the brain.

According to another theory, some experts in acupuncture claim that acupuncture helps the patient's body transmit signals via the fascia. The fascia is a band of connective tissues located beneath the skin. It surrounds all body muscles. Some acupuncturists claim that the body's meridians are myofascial chains and that is why the effects of stimulating an acupuncture point in the lower leg may affect other parts of the body.

How to Prepare for Acupuncture

There are no special procedures to take before acupuncture treatment. However, you need to choose a reliable practitioner who knows how to perform the procedure. Take the following steps to find the best acupuncture practitioner:

- Look for advice and recommendations from the people you trust.
- Examine the practitioner's credentials and experience. In most countries, nonphysician acupuncturists are required to pass an examination conducted by the relevant medical organization or government body. Additionally, most states require registration, certification, or license. A license may not guarantee quality services, but it shows that the practitioner meets the necessary standards and knows how to perform the procedure.
- Schedule and conduct an interview with the selected acupuncture practitioner. Remember to ask them how the procedure is done, the possible health benefits depending on your health condition, how much you are required to pay, and the estimated number of treatments. A good practitioner will tell you the success rate of using the procedure.
- If you want to pay through insurance, find out whether your insurer covers the procedure.

You should also consider other factors if you choose acupuncture as an alternative treatment option. For instance, you should never replace professional health care with acupuncture or postpone your appointment with a doctor because you are using acupuncture. You should also bear in mind that some conventional healthcare providers including dentists and physicians practice acupuncture.

Conclusion

This book has explored the origins of acupuncture and explained its health benefits and the possible side effects. According to various historians, the practice of acupuncture may have been around for many centuries based on evidence from ancient Chinese texts, tombs, and other places. Over the years, the practice has experienced major changes because of traditional beliefs, cultural practices, and scientific research. Some people may say that acupuncture has no health benefits because it seems to be an ancient health practice. However, evidence from scientific research has revealed that those suffering from certain health problems may benefit from acupuncture in different ways. The practice has been integrated into the modern healthcare system because of positive results from scientific studies and the experiences of acupuncture users.

Even though acupuncture was first practiced in China, the practice has spread to Western countries and other parts of the world. Many people in different countries can now enjoy the benefits of this alternative treatment method. Some health insurers have even offered to provide coverage to those willing to use acupuncture services. Governments have also issued licenses to acupuncturists and medical doctors who have undergone the necessary training. Many people have benefited from the practice and research shows that the number of people who use acupuncture has continued to increase over the years.

For many years, people have used acupuncture to prevent and cure a wide range of health problems. Patients who have benefited from the practice include those suffering from pains and aches in different parts of the body. Besides relieving pain, acupuncture may treat the underlying health problem. The best part is that acupuncture can improve your overall well-being by manipulating the body's energy (chi) and energy points.

Since there are many practitioners offering acupuncture services today, you need to pay attention to the recommended safety measures. It is also important to ensure that your provider has the required training and license. Also, make sure your acupuncturist uses new and sterilized needles in each session to avoid infections and other health problems.

Just like other treatment options and health practices, there are significant issues regarding the use of acupuncture as an alternative treatment option. Acupuncture may be considered to be a traditional or cultural health practice with no health benefits, but the results have proven that it can be useful when used to treat specific health conditions. Many acupuncture users have told the world about the benefits of the procedure and scientific research shows that those suffering from certain illnesses may benefit from it. You should probably try the procedure if you have been suffering from pains and aches. Remember to contact your doctor to learn about the possible benefits and risks.